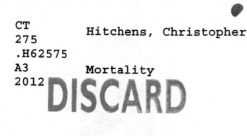

Mortality

Mortality

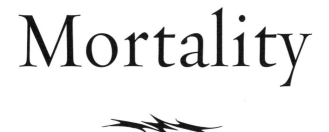

Christopher Hitchens

Foreword by Graydon Carter
Afterword by Carol Blue

TWELVE

NEW YORK   BOSTON

Twelve

Hachette Book Group

237 Park Avenue

New York, NY 10017

www.HachetteBookGroup.com

Printed in the United States of America

RRD-C

First Edition: September 2012

10 9 8 7 6 5 4 3 2 1

Twelve is an imprint of Grand Central Publishing.
The Twelve name and logo are trademarks of Hachette Book Group, Inc.

The Hachette Speakers Bureau provides a wide range of authors for speaking events. To find out more, go to www.hachettespeakersbureau.com or call (866) 376-6591.

The publisher is not responsible for websites (or their content) that are not owned by the publisher.

Library of Congress Cataloging-in-Publication Data
Hitchens, Christopher.
Mortality / Christopher Hitchens. — 1st ed.
p. cm.
Summary: "Courageous, insightful and candid thoughts on malady and mortality from one of our most celebrated writers"—Provided by the publisher.
ISBN 978-1-4555-0275-2 (regular ed.)
1. Hitchens, Christopher—Health. 2. Cancer—Patients—United States—Biography. 3. Terminally ill—United States—Biography.
4. Mortality. 5. Death. 6. Authors, American—Biography. I. Title.
CT275.H62575A3 2012
304.6'4—dc23
2012014024

Grateful acknowledgment is made to Vanity Fair, *in which much of this book first appeared, in somewhat different form.*

FOREWORD BY GRAYDON CARTER

At a dinner in Los Angeles this spring, a young actor named Emile Hirsch came up to me in a state of high excitement. He knew I had worked with Christopher Hitchens for many years, and he just wanted to talk about Christopher with someone who knew him. He'd read *Hitch-22* and was well into the Kissinger book, and he said that Christopher's writing had affected him in a way that almost no one else's had. In the months following Christopher's death, I had similar encounters with young people who felt compelled to talk about how his writing had touched them. It's no exaggeration to say that Christopher had few equals in the sphere of spirited commentary. But there was something in his saucy fearlessness, in his great turbine of a mind, and in his sociable but unpredictable brand of anarchy that seriously touched kids in their twenties and early thirties in much the same way that Hunter S. Thompson had a generation before. Young Emile asked if there was going to be a memorial service, and I told him that there would be one in New York and that we were bookmarking April 20th as a tentative date.

The memorial was indeed held on the 20th, in the Great Hall at Cooper Union in Greenwich Village. My *Vanity Fair* colleagues Aimée Bell (Christopher's longtime editor at the magazine) and Sara Marks organized the readings—all of them from Christopher's own work. We wanted to produce a program that would be cozy and loving, but in no way sentimental or mawkish. And the great and the good of English letters turned up to pay tribute—and to console his widow, Carol, and his three children. Martin Amis, Tom Stoppard, Salman Rushdie, Ian McEwan, and James Fenton were there and they all spoke. Editors such as Anna Wintour, David Remnick, Jim Kelly, and Rick Stengel came; so did Christopher's brother Peter, Andrew Sullivan, Christopher Buckley, Andrew and Leslie Cockburn and their daughter the fine actress Olivia Wilde, and Andrew's brother Patrick. The Bush administration was represented by former deputy defense secretary Paul Wolfowitz—a remnant of the curious right turn Christopher took in the lead-up to the Iraq War. Hollywood was represented by Sean Penn—and, as I was pleased to see, by young Mr. Hirsch.

After the memorial, the participants retired to the Waverly Inn nearby and drank and smoked in the sunshine and reminisced about Christopher. Although the day was bathed in sorrow, there was a magical quality to the afternoon as it spilled into the evening and through to midnight, when there were still a dozen or more mourners. For those who were there, Christopher's memorial was, as we used to say in the 1960s, a happening, and a day we will not soon forget.

For the fact is that Christopher was one of life's singular characters—a wit, a charmer, a troublemaker, and a dear and devoted friend. He was a man of insatiable appetites—for cigarettes, for scotch, for company, for great writing, and, above all, for conversation. That he had an output to equal what he took in was the miracle in the man. You'd be hard-pressed to find a writer who could match the outpouring of exquisitely crafted columns, essays, articles, and books he produced over the past four decades. He wrote often—constantly, in fact, and right up to the end. And Christopher wrote fast, frequently without the benefit of a second draft or even corrections. Perhaps in the back of his mind he knew that his time on the stage would end in the second act, and he was racing to get it all in, and to get it all out. I can recall a lunch in 1991, when I was editing the *New York Observer*, and he and Aimée and I got together for a quick bite at a restaurant on Madison, no longer there. Christopher's copy was due early that afternoon. Pre-lunch tumblers of scotch were followed by a couple of glasses of wine during the meal and then a couple of post-meal cognacs. That was *his* intake. After stumbling back to the office, we set him up at a rickety table and an old Olivetti, and in a symphony of clacking he produced a 1,000-word column of near perfection in under half an hour.

Christopher was one of the first writers I called when I came to *Vanity Fair*, in 1992. Six years before, I had asked him to write for *Spy*. That offer was politely rejected. The *Vanity Fair* approach had a fee attached, though, and to my everlasting credit, he accepted and was the signature columnist for the magazine from then on. With the exception of Dominick Dunne (who died in 2009), no writer has been more associated with *Vanity Fair.* There was no subject too big or too small for Christopher. Over the past two decades he traveled to just about every hot spot you can think of. He also subjected himself to any manner of humiliation or discomfort in the name of his column. I once sent him out on a mission to break the most niggling laws still on the books in New York City, one of which forbade riding a bicycle with your feet off the pedals. The photograph that ran with the column, of Christopher sailing a small bike through Central Park with his legs in the air, looked like something out of the Moscow Circus. At the suggestion of Tom Hedley, an old hand from Harold Hayes's *Esquire,* I set him off on a course of self-improvement for a three-part series, in which he would subject himself to myriad treatments to refurbish his dental area and other dark regions. At one point I suggested he go to a well-regarded waxing parlor in town for what they indelicately call the "sack, back, and crack." He struggled to absorb the full meaning of this, but after a few seconds he smiled a nervous smile and said, "In for a penny…"

Christopher was the beau ideal of the public intellectual. You felt as though he was writing to you and to you alone. And as a result many readers felt they knew him. Walking with him down the street in New York or through an airplane terminal was like escorting a movie star through the throngs. Christopher was not just brave in facing the illness that took him but brave in words and thought. He did not mind landing outside the cozy cocoon of conventional liberal wisdom, his pro-war stance before the invasion of Iraq being but one example. Friends distanced themselves from him during those unlit days. But he stuck to his guns. After his rather famous 1995 attack on Mother Teresa, one of our contributing editors, a devout Catholic, came into the office filled with umbrage and announced that he was canceling his subscription. "You can't cancel it," I said. "You get the magazine for free." Years ago, in the midst of the Clinton impeachment uproar, Christopher had a very public dustup with his friend Sidney Blumenthal, a Clinton White House functionary—the dispute was over which part of a conversation between them was or was not on the record. Christopher wound up on television a lot defending himself. He looked like hell, and I suggested we bring him to New York for a bit of a makeover and some R&R away from the cameras. The magazine was pretty flush back then, and we set him up with a new suit, shirts, ties, and such. When someone from the fashion department asked him what size his shoes were, he said he didn't know— the pair he had on was borrowed.

I could not begin to list the pantheon of public intellectuals and close friends who will mourn his passing, and it is not limited to those who made it to his memorial. Christopher had his share of lady admirers too, including—but certainly not limited to—Ms. Wintour, back when he was young and still relatively fragrant. His wife, Carol, a writer, filmmaker, and legendary hostess, set a high bar in how to handle a flower like Christopher, both when he was healthy and during his more weakened days. An invitation to their vast apartment in the Wyoming, on Columbia Road in Washington, D.C., was a prized reward for being a part of their circle or even on the fringes of it. We used to hold an anti–White

House Correspondents' Dinner party there in the 1990s and 2000s; the Salon des Refusés, he called it. You could meet anyone there. From Supreme Court justices to right-wing windbags to, well, Barbra Streisand and other assorted totems of the left. He was a good friend who wished his friends well. And as a result he had a lot of them.

Christopher had an enviable career arc that began with his own brand of fiery journalism at Britain's *New Statesman* and then wended its way to America, where he wrote for everyone from the *Atlantic* and *Harper's* to *Slate* and the *New York Times Book Review*. And we all called him our own. He was a legend on the speakers' circuit and could debate just about anyone on anything. He won umpteen awards (although that was not the sort of thing that fueled his work) and in the last decade he wrote best-sellers, including his well-received, best-selling memoir, *Hitch-22,* that finally put some money into his family's pocket. In the last weeks of his life, he was told that an asteroid had been named after him. He was pleased by the thought, and inasmuch as the word is derived from the Greek, meaning "star-like," and asteroids are known to be volatile, it is a fitting honor.

To his friends, Christopher will be remembered for his elevated but inclusive humor and for a staggering, almost punishing memory that held up under the most liquid of late-night conditions. And to all of us, his readers, Christopher Hitchens will be remembered for the words he left behind. These last ones, free as they are of sentiment or self-pity, are among his last. They are also among his best.

June 2012
New York City

Mortality

I

I HAVE MORE THAN ONCE IN MY TIME WOKEN UP feeling like death. But nothing prepared me for the early morning in June when I came to consciousness feeling as if I were actually shackled to my own corpse. The whole cave of my chest and thorax seemed to have been hollowed out and then refilled with slow-drying cement. I could faintly hear myself breathe but could not manage to inflate my lungs. My heart was beating either much too much or much too little. Any movement, however slight, required forethought and planning. It took strenuous effort for me to cross the room of my New York hotel and summon the emergency services.

They arrived with great dispatch and behaved with immense courtesy and professionalism. I had the time to wonder why they needed so many boots and helmets and so much heavy backup equipment, but now that I view the scene in retrospect I see it as a very gentle and firm deportation, taking me from the country of the well across the stark frontier that marks off the land of malady. Within a few hours, having had to do quite a lot of emergency work on my heart and my lungs, the physicians at this sad border post had shown me a few other postcards from the interior and told me that my immediate next stop would have to be with an oncologist. Some kind of shadow was throwing itself across the negatives.

The previous evening, I had been launching my latest book at a successful event in New Haven. The night of the terrible morning, I was supposed to go on *The Daily Show* with Jon Stewart and then appear at a sold-out event at the 92nd Street Y, on the Upper East Side, in conversation with Salman Rushdie. My very short-lived campaign of denial took this form: I would not cancel these appearances or let down my friends or miss the chance of selling a stack of books. I managed to pull off both gigs without anyone noticing anything amiss, though I did vomit two times, with an extraordinary combination of accuracy, neatness, violence, and profusion, just before each show. This is what citizens of the sick country do while they are still hopelessly clinging to their old domicile.

The new land is quite welcoming in its way. Everybody smiles encouragingly and there appears to be absolutely no racism. A generally egalitarian spirit prevails, and those who run the place have obviously got where they are on merit and hard work. As against that, the humor is a touch feeble and repetitive, there seems to be almost no talk of sex, and the cuisine is the worst of any destination I have ever visited. The country has a language of its own—a lingua franca that manages to be both dull and difficult and that contains names like ondansetron, for anti-nausea medication—as well as some unsettling gestures that require a bit of getting used to. For example, an official met for the first time may abruptly sink his fingers into your neck. That's how I discovered that my cancer had spread to my lymph nodes, and that one of these deformed beauties—located on my right clavicle, or collarbone—was big enough to be seen and felt. It's not at all good when your cancer is "palpable" from the outside. Especially when, as at this stage, they didn't even know where the primary source was. Carcinoma works cunningly from the inside out. Detection and treatment often work more slowly and gropingly, from the outside in. Many needles were sunk into my clavicle area—"Tissue is the issue" being a hot slogan in the local Tumorville tongue—and I was told the biopsy results might take a week.

Working back from the cancer-ridden squamous cells that these first results disclosed, it took rather longer than that to discover the disagreeable truth. The word "metastasized" was the one in the report that first caught my eye, and ear. The alien had colonized a bit of my lung as well as quite a bit of my lymph node. And its original base of operations was located—had been located for quite some time—in my esophagus. My father had died, and very swiftly, too, of cancer of the esophagus. He was seventy-nine. I am sixty-one. In whatever kind of a "race" life may be, I have very abruptly become a finalist.

The notorious stage theory of Elisabeth Kübler-Ross, whereby one progresses from denial to rage through bargaining to depression and the eventual bliss of "acceptance," hasn't so far had much application to my case. In one way, I suppose, I have been "in denial" for some time, knowingly burning the candle at both ends and finding that it often gives a lovely light. But for precisely that reason, I can't see myself smiting my brow with shock or hear myself whining about how it's all so unfair: I have been taunting the Reaper into taking a free scythe in my direction and have now succumbed to something so predictable and banal that it bores even me. Rage would be beside the point for the same reason. Instead, I am badly oppressed by the gnawing sense of waste. I had real plans for my next decade and felt I'd worked hard enough to earn it. Will I really not live to see my children married? To watch the World Trade Center rise again? To read—if not indeed to write—the obituaries of elderly villains like Henry Kissinger and Joseph Ratzinger? But I understand this sort of non-thinking for what it is: sentimentality and self-pity. Of course my book hit the bestseller list on the day that I received the grimmest of news bulletins, and for that matter the last flight I took as a healthy-feeling person (to a fine, big audience at the Chicago Book Fair) was the one that made me a million-miler on United Airlines, with a lifetime of free upgrades to look forward to. But irony is my business and I just can't see any ironies here: Would it be less poignant to get cancer on the day that my memoirs were remaindered as a box-office turkey, or that I was bounced from a coach-class flight and left on the tarmac? To the dumb question "Why me?" the cosmos barely bothers to return the reply: Why not?

The *bargaining* stage, though. Maybe there's a loophole here. The oncology bargain is that, in return for at least the chance of a few more useful years, you agree to submit to chemotherapy and then, if you are lucky with that, to radiation or even surgery. So here's the wager: You stick around for a bit, but in return we are going to need some things from you. These things may include your taste buds, your ability to concentrate, your ability to digest, and the hair on your head. This certainly appears to be a reasonable trade. Unfortunately, it also involves confronting one of the most appealing clichés in our language. You've heard it all right. People don't have cancer: They are reported to be battling cancer. No well-wisher omits the combative image: You can beat this. It's even in obituaries for cancer losers, as if one might reasonably say of someone that they died after a long and brave struggle with mortality. You don't hear it about long-term sufferers from heart disease or kidney failure.

Myself, I love the imagery of struggle. I sometimes wish I were suffering in a good cause, or risking my life for the good of others, instead of just being a gravely endangered patient. Allow me to inform you, though, that when you sit in a room with a set of other finalists, and kindly people bring a huge transparent bag of poison and plug it into your arm, and you either read or don't read a book while the venom sack gradually empties itself into your system, the image of the ardent soldier or revolutionary is the very last one that will occur to you. You feel swamped with passivity and impotence: dissolving in powerlessness like a sugar lump in water.

It's quite something, this chemo-poison. It has caused me to lose about fourteen pounds, though without making me feel any lighter. It has cleared up a vicious rash on my shins that no doctor could ever name, let alone cure. (Some venom, to get rid of those furious red dots without a struggle.) Let it please be this mean and ruthless with the alien and its spreading dead-zone colonies. But as against that, the death-dealing stuff and life-preserving stuff have also made me strangely neuter. I was fairly reconciled to the loss of my hair, which began to come out in the shower in the first two weeks of treatment, and which I saved in a plastic bag so that it could help fill a floating dam in the Gulf of Mexico. But I wasn't quite prepared for the way that my razor blade would suddenly go slipping pointlessly down my face, meeting no stubble. Or for the way that my newly smooth upper lip would begin to look as if it had undergone electrolysis, causing me to look a bit too much like somebody's maiden auntie. (The chest hair that was once the toast of two continents hasn't yet wilted, but so much of it was shaved off for various hospital incisions that it's a rather patchy affair.) I feel upsettingly denatured. If Penélope Cruz were one of my nurses, I wouldn't even notice. In the war against Thanatos, if we must term it a war, the immediate loss of Eros is a huge initial sacrifice.

These are my first raw reactions to being stricken. I am quietly resolved to resist bodily as best I can, even if only passively, and to seek the most advanced advice. My heart and blood pressure and many other registers are now strong again: Indeed, it occurs to me that if I didn't have such a stout constitution I might have led a much healthier life thus far. Against me is the blind, emotionless alien, cheered on by some who have long wished me ill. But on the side of my continued life is a group of brilliant and selfless physicians plus an astonishing number of prayer groups. On both of these I hope to write next time if—as my father invariably said— I am spared.

II

WHEN I DESCRIBED THE TUMOR IN MY ESOPHAGUS as a "blind, emotionless alien," I suppose that even I couldn't help awarding it some of the qualities of a living thing. This at least I know to be a mistake: an instance of the pathetic fallacy (angry cloud, proud mountain, presumptuous little Beaujolais) by which we ascribe animate qualities to inanimate phenomena. To exist, a cancer needs a living organism, but it cannot ever *become* a living organism. Its whole malice—there I go again—lies in the fact that the "best" it can do is to die with its host. Either that or its host will find the measures with which to extirpate and outlive it.

But, as I knew before I became ill, there are some people for whom this explanation is unsatisfying. To them, a rodent carcinoma really is a dedicated, conscious agent—a slow-acting suicide-murderer—on a consecrated mission from heaven. You haven't lived, if I can put it like this, until you have read contributions such as this on the websites of the faithful:

> Who else feels Christopher Hitchens getting terminal throat cancer [*sic*] was God's revenge for him using his voice to blaspheme him? Atheists like to ignore FACTS. They like to act like everything is a "coincidence." Really? It's just a "coincidence" [that] out of any part of his body, Christopher Hitchens got cancer in the one part of his body he used for blasphemy? Yeah, keep believing that, Atheists. He's going to writhe in agony and pain and wither away to nothing and then die a horrible agonizing death, and THEN comes the real fun, when he's sent to HELLFIRE forever to be tortured and set afire.

There are numerous passages in holy scripture and religious tradition that for centuries made this kind of gloating into a mainstream belief. Long before it concerned me particularly I had understood the obvious objections. First, which mere primate is so damn sure that he can know the mind of god? Second, would this anonymous author want his views to be read by my unoffending children, who are also being given a hard time in their way, and by the same god? Third, why not a thunderbolt for yours truly, or something similarly awe-inspiring? The vengeful deity has a sadly depleted arsenal if all he can think of is exactly the cancer that my age and former "lifestyle" would suggest that I got. Fourth, why cancer at all? Almost all men get cancer of the prostate if they live long enough: It's an undignified thing but quite evenly distributed among saints and sinners, believers and unbelievers. If you maintain that god awards the appropriate cancers, you must also account for the numbers of infants who contract leukemia. Devout persons have died young and in pain. Betrand Russell and Voltaire, by contrast, remained spry until the end, as many psychopathic criminals and tyrants have also done. These visitations, then, seem awfully random. My so far uncancerous throat, let me rush to assure my Christian correspondent above, is not *at all* the only organ with which I have blasphemed. And even if my voice goes before I do, I shall continue to write polemics against religious delusions, at least until it's hello darkness my old friend. In which case, why not cancer of the brain? As a terrified, half-aware imbecile, I might even scream for a priest at the close of business, though I hereby state while I am still lucid that the entity thus humiliating itself would not in fact be "me." (Bear this in mind, in case of any later rumors or fabrications.)

The absorbing fact about being mortally sick is that you spend a good deal of time preparing yourself to die with some modicum of stoicism (and provision for loved ones), while being simultaneously and highly interested in the business of survival. This is a distinctly bizarre way of "living"—lawyers in the morning and doctors in the afternoon—and means that one has to exist even more than usual in a double frame of mind. The same is true, it seems, of those who pray for me. And most of these are just as "religious" as the chap who wants me to be tortured in the here and now—which I will be even if I eventually recover—and then tortured forever into the bargain if I *don't* recover or, presumably and ultimately, even if I do.

Of the astonishing and flattering number of people who wrote to me when I fell so ill, very few failed to say one of two things. Either they assured me that they wouldn't offend me by offering prayers or they tenderly insisted that they would pray anyway. Devotional websites consecrated special space to the question. (If you should read this in time, by all means keep in mind that September 20, 2010, has already been designated "Everybody Pray for Hitchens Day.") Pat Archbold, at the *National Catholic Register*, and Deacon Greg Kandra were among the Roman Catholics who thought me a worthy object of prayer. Rabbi David Wolpe, author of *Why Faith Matters* and the leader of a major congregation in Los Angeles, said the same. He has been a debating partner of mine, as have several Protestant evangelical conservatives like Pastor Douglas Wilson of the New Saint Andrews College and Larry Taunton of the Fixed Point Foundation in Birmingham, Alabama. Both wrote to say that their assemblies were praying for me. And it was to them that it first occurred to me to write back, asking: Praying for what?

As with many of the Catholics who essentially pray for me to see the light as much as to get better, they were very honest. Salvation was the main point. "We are, to be sure, concerned for your health, too, but that is a very secondary consideration. 'For what shall it profit a man if he gains the whole world and forfeits his own soul?' [Matthew 16:26]." That was Larry Taunton. Pastor Wilson responded that when he heard the news he prayed for three things: that I would fight off the disease, that I would make myself right with eternity, and that the process would bring the two of us back into contact. He couldn't resist adding rather puckishly that the third prayer had already been answered...

So there are some quite reputable Catholics, Jews, and Protestants who think that I might in some sense of the word be worth saving. The Muslim faction has been quieter. An Iranian friend has asked for a prayer to be said for me at the grave of Omar Khayyam, supreme poet of Persian freethinkers. The YouTube video announcing the day of intercession for me is accompanied by the song "I Think I See the Light," performed by the same Cat Stevens who as "Yusuf Islam" once endorsed the hysterical

Iranian theocratic call to murder my friend Salman Rushdie. (The banal lyrics of his pseudo-uplifting song, by the way, appear to be addressed to a chick.) And this apparent ecumenism has other contradictions, too. If I were to announce that I had suddenly converted to Catholicism, I know that Larry Taunton and Douglas Wilson would feel I had fallen into grievous error. On the other hand, if I were to join either of their Protestant evangelical groups, the followers of Rome would not think my soul was much safer than it is now, while a late-in-life decision to adhere to Judaism or Islam would inevitably lose me many prayers from both factions. I sympathize afresh with the mighty Voltaire, who, when badgered on his deathbed and urged to renounce the devil, murmured that this was no time to be making enemies.

The Danish physicist and Nobelist Niels Bohr once hung a horseshoe over his doorway. Appalled friends exclaimed that surely he didn't put any trust in such pathetic superstition. "No, I don't," he replied with composure, "but apparently it works whether you believe in it or not." That might be the safest conclusion. The most comprehensive investigation of the subject ever conducted—the "Study of the Therapeutic Effects of Intercessory Prayer," of 2006, could find no correlation at all between the number and regularity of prayers offered and the likelihood that the person being prayed for would have improved chances. But it did find a small but interesting *negative* correlation, in that some patients suffered slight additional woe when they failed to manifest any improvement. They felt that they had disappointed their devoted supporters. And morale is another unquantifiable factor in survival. I now understand this better than I did when I first read it. An enormous number of secular and atheist friends have told me encouraging and flattering things like, "If anyone can beat this, you can"; "Cancer has no chance against someone like you"; "We know you can vanquish this." On bad days, and even on better ones, such exhortations can have a vaguely depressing effect. If I check out, I'll be letting all these comrades down. A different secular problem also occurs to me: What if I pulled through and the pious faction contentedly claimed that their prayers had been answered? That would somehow be irritating.

I have saved the best of the faithful until the last. Dr. Francis Collins is one of the greatest living Americans. He is the man who brought the Human Genome Project to completion, ahead of time and under budget, and who now directs the National Institutes of Health. In his work on the genetic origins of disorder, he helped decode the "misprints" that cause such calamities as cystic fibrosis and Huntington's disease. He is working now on the amazing healing properties that are latent in stem cells and in "targeted" gene-based treatments. This great humanitarian is also a devotee of the work of C. S. Lewis and in his book *The Language of God* has set out the case for making science compatible with faith. (This small volume contains an admirably terse chapter informing fundamentalists that the argument about evolution is over, mainly because there *is* no argument.) I know Francis, too, from various public and private debates over religion. He has been kind enough to visit me in his own time and to discuss all sorts of novel treatments, only recently even imaginable, that might apply to my case. And let me put it this way: He hasn't suggested prayer, and I in turn haven't teased him about *The Screwtape*

Letters. So those who want me to die in agony are really praying that the efforts of our most selfless Christian physician be thwarted. Who is Dr. Collins to interfere with the divine design? By a similar twist, those who want me to burn in hell are also mocking those kind religious folk who do not find me unsalvageably evil. I leave these paradoxes to those, friends and enemies, who still venerate the supernatural.

Pursuing the prayer thread through the labyrinth of the Web, I eventually found a bizarre "Place Bets" video. This invites potential punters to put money on whether I will repudiate my atheism and embrace religion by a certain date or continue to affirm unbelief and take the hellish consequences. This isn't, perhaps, as cheap or as nasty as it may sound. One of Christianity's most cerebral defenders, Blaise Pascal, reduced the essentials to a wager as far back as the seventeenth century. Put your faith in the almighty, he proposed, and you stand to gain everything. Decline the heavenly offer and you lose everything if the coin falls the other way. (Some philosophers also call this Pascal's Gambit.)

Ingenious though the full reasoning of his essay may be—he was one of the founders of probability theory—Pascal assumes both a cynical god and an abjectly opportunist human being. Suppose I ditch the principles I have held for a lifetime, in the hope of gaining favor at the last minute? I hope and trust that no serious person would be at all impressed by such a hucksterish choice. Meanwhile, the god who would reward cowardice and dishonesty and punish irreconcilable doubt is among the many gods in which (whom?) I do not believe. I don't mean to be churlish about any kind intentions, but when September 20 comes, please do not trouble deaf heaven with your bootless cries. Unless, of course, it makes *you* feel better.

Many readers are familiar with the spirit and the letter of the definition of "prayer," as given by Ambrose Bierce in his *Devil's Dictionary*. It runs like this, and is extremely easy to comprehend:

> Prayer: A petition that the laws of nature be suspended in favor of the petitioner; himself confessedly unworthy.

Everybody can see the joke that is lodged within this entry: The man who prays is the one who thinks that god has arranged matters all wrong, but who also thinks that he can instruct god how to put them right. Half-buried in the contradiction is the distressing idea that nobody is in charge, or nobody with any moral authority. The call to prayer is self-cancelling. Those of us who don't take part in it will justify our abstention on the grounds that we do not need, or care, to undergo the futile process of continuous reinforcement. Either our convictions are enough in themselves or they are not: At any rate they do require standing in a crowd and uttering constant and uniform incantations. This is ordered by one religion to take place five times a day, and by other monotheists for almost that number, while all of them set aside at least one whole day for the exclusive praise of the Lord, and Judaism seems to consist in its original constitution of a huge list of prohibitions that must be followed before all else.

The tone of the prayers replicates the silliness of the mandate, in that god is enjoined or thanked to do what he was going to do anyway. Thus the Jewish male begins each day by thanking god for not making him into a woman (or a Gentile), while the Jewish woman contents herself with thanking the almighty for creating her "as she is." Presumably the almighty is pleased to receive this tribute to his power and the approval of those he created. It's just that, if he is truly almighty, the achievement would seem rather a slight one.

Much the same applies to the idea that prayer, instead of making Christianity look foolish, makes it appear convincing. (We'll just stay with Christianity today.) Now, it can be asserted with some confidence, first, that its deity is all-wise and all-powerful and, second, that its congregants stand in desperate need of that deity's infinite wisdom and power. Just to give some elementary quotations, it is stated in the book of Philippians, 4:6, "Be careful for nothing; but in everything by prayer and supplication and thanksgiving, let your requests be known to God." Deuteronomy 32:4 proclaims that "he is the rock, his work is perfect," and Isaiah 64:8 tells us, "Now O Lord, thou art our father; we art clay and thou our potter; and we are all the work of thy hand." Note, then, that Christianity insists on the absolute dependence of its flock, and then only on the offering of undiluted praise and thanks. A person using prayer time to ask for the world to be set to rights, or to beseech god to bestow a favor upon himself, would in effect be guilty of a profound blasphemy or at the very least a pathetic misunderstanding. It is not for the mere human to be presuming that he or she can advise the divine. And this, sad to say, opens religion to the additional charge of corruption. The leaders of the church know perfectly well that prayer is not intended to gratify the devout. So that, every time they accept a donation in return for some petition, they are accepting a gross negation of their faith: a faith that depends on the passive acceptance of the devout and not on their making demands for betterment. Eventually, and after a bitter and schismatic quarrel, practices like the notorious "sale of indulgences" were abandoned. But many a fine basilica or chantry would not be standing today if this awful violation had *not* turned such a spectacularly good profit.

And today it is easy enough to see, at the revival meetings of Protestant fundamentalists, the counting of the checks and bills before the laying on of hands by the preacher has even been completed. Again, the spectacle is a shameless one, with the Calvinists having in some ways replaced Rome as the most exorbitant holy fund-raisers. And—before we run out of contradictions—it seems doubly absurd for a Calvinist to take an interest in divine intercession. The founding constitution of the Presbyterian Church famously proclaimed from Philadelphia that "by the decree of God, for the manifestation of his glory, some men and angels are predestinated unto everlasting life and others fore-ordained for everlasting death...without any foresight of faith or good works, or perseverance in either of them, or any other thing in the creature, as conditions." Plainly put, this means that it does not matter whether you try to lead a holy life, or even succeed in doing so. Random caprice will still determine whether or not you receive a heavenly reward. In these circumstances, the emptiness of prayer is almost the least of it. Beyond that minor futility, the religion which treats its flock as a credulous plaything offers one of the cruelest spectacles that can be imagined: a human being in fear and doubt who is openly exploited to believe in the impossible. In the argument over prayer, then, please do not be shocked if it is we atheists who wear the pitying look as any moment of moral crisis threatens to draw near.

III

I figure she should take care of herself, put herself in a deep freeze, and in a year or two in all likelihood they'll develop a pill that'll clear this up simple as a common cold. Already, you know, some of these cortisones; but the doctor tells us they don't know but what the side effects may be worse. You know: the big C. My figuring is, take the chance, they're just about ready to lick cancer anyway and with these transplants pretty soon they can replace your whole insides.

—Mr. Angstrom Sr. in John Updike's
Rabbit Redux (1971)

UPDIKE'S NOVEL WAS SET IN WHAT MIGHT BE called the optimistic years of the Nixon administration: the time of the Apollo mission and the birth of that all-American can-do expression that begins, "If we can put a man on the moon…" In January 1971, Senators Kennedy and Javits sponsored the "Conquest of Cancer Act," and by December of that year Richard Nixon had signed something like it into law, along with huge federal appropriations. The talk was all of a "War on Cancer."

Four decades later, those other glorious "wars," on poverty and drugs and terror, combine to mock such rhetoric, and, as often as I am encouraged to "battle" my own tumor, I can't shake the feeling that it is the cancer that is making war on me. The dread with which it is discussed—"the big C"—is still almost superstitious. So is the ever whispered hope of a new treatment or cure.

In her famous essay on Hollywood, Pauline Kael described it as a place where you could die of encouragement. That may still be true of Tinseltown; in Tumortown you sometimes feel that you may expire from sheer *advice*. A lot of it comes free and unsolicited. I must, without delay, begin ingesting the granulated essence of the peach pit (or is it the apricot?), a sovereign remedy known to ancient civilizations but now covered up by greedy modern doctors. Another correspondent urges heaping doses of testosterone supplements, perhaps as a morale-booster. Or I must find ways of opening certain chakras and putting myself in an appropriately receptive mental state. Macrobiotic or vegan diets will be all I require for nourishment during this experience. And don't laugh at poor old Mr. Angstrom above: Somebody has written to me from a famous university to suggest that I have myself cryonically or cryogenically frozen against the day when the magic bullet, or whatever it is, has been devised. (When I failed to reply to this, I got a second missive, suggesting that I freeze at least my brain so that its cortex could be appreciated by posterity. Well, I mean to say, gosh, thanks awfully.) As against all that, I did get a kind note from a Cheyenne-Arapaho friend of mine, saying that everyone she knew who had resorted to tribal remedies had died almost immediately, and suggesting that if I was offered any Native American medicines I should "move as fast as possible in the opposite direction." Some advice can actually be taken.

Even in the world of sanity and modernity, though, it often cannot. Extremely well-informed people also get in touch to insist that there is really only one doctor, or only one clinic. These physicians and facilities are as far apart as Cleveland and Kyoto. Even if I had possession of my own aircraft, I would never be able to assure myself that I had tried everyone, let alone everything. The citizens of Tumortown are forever assailed with cures, and rumors of cures. I actually did take myself to one grand *palazzo* of a clinic in the richer part of the stricken city, which I will not name because all I got from it was a long and dull exposition of what I already knew plus (while lying on one of the fabled establishment's examination tables) a bugbite that briefly doubled the size of my left hand: completely surplus even to my pre-cancerous requirements but a real irritation to someone with a chemically corroded immune system.

Still and all, this is both an exhilarating and a melancholy time to have a cancer like mine. Exhilarating, because my calm and scholarly oncologist, Dr. Frederick Smith, can design a chemo-cocktail that has already shrunk some of my secondary tumors, and can "tweak" said cocktail to minimize certain nasty side effects. That wouldn't have been possible when Updike was writing his book or when Nixon was proclaiming his "war." But melancholy, too, because new peaks of medicine are rising and new treatments beginning to be glimpsed, and they have probably come too late for me.

For example, I was encouraged to learn of a new "immunotherapy protocol," evolved by Drs. Steven Rosenberg and Nicholas Restifo at the National Cancer Institute. Actually, the word "encouraged" is an understatement. I was hugely excited. It is now possible to remove T cells from the blood, subject them to a process of genetic engineering, and then reinject them to attack the malignancy. "Some of this may sound like space-age medicine," wrote Dr. Restifo, as if he, too, had been rereading Updike, "but we have treated well over 100 patients with gene-engineered T cells, and have treated over 20 patients with the exact approach that I am suggesting may be applicable to your case." There was a catch, and it involved a "match." My tumor had to express a protein called NY-ESO-1, and my immune cells had to have a particular molecule named HLA-A2. Given this pairing, the immune system could be charged up to resist the tumor. The odds looked good, in that half of those with European or Caucasian genes do have that very molecule. And my tumor when analyzed did have the protein! But my immune cells declined to identify as sufficiently "Caucasian." Other similar trials are under review by the Food and Drug Administration, but I am in a bit of a hurry, and I can't forget the feeling of flatness that I experienced when I received the news.

Best perhaps to get these false hopes behind one quickly: It was in the same week that I was told that I didn't have the necessary mutations in my tumor to qualify for any other of the "targeted" cancer therapies currently on offer. A night or so later I was emailed by perhaps fifty friends because *60 Minutes* had run a segment about the "tissue engineering," by way of stem cells, of a man with a cancerous esophagus. He had effectively been medically enabled to "grow" a new one. I excitedly contacted my friend Dr. Collins, father of genome-based treatment, who gently but firmly told me that my cancer has spread too far beyond my esophagus to be treatable by such a means.

Analyzing the blues that I developed during those lousy seven days, I discovered that I felt cheated as well as disappointed. "Until you have done something for humanity," wrote the great American educator Horace Mann, "you should be ashamed to die." I would have happily offered myself as an experimental subject for new drugs or new surgeries, partly of course in the hope that they might salvage me, but also on the Mann principle. And I didn't even qualify for the adventure. So I have to trudge on with the chemo routine, augmented if it proves worthwhile by radiation and perhaps the much-discussed CyberKnife for a surgical intervention: both of these things near-miraculous when compared with the recent past.

There is an even longer shot that I do propose to attempt, even though its likely efficacy lies at the outer limits of probability. I am going to try to have my entire DNA "sequenced," along with the genome of my tumor. Francis Collins was typically sober in his evaluation of the usefulness of this. If the two sequencings could be performed, he wrote to me, "it could be clearly determined what mutations were present in the cancer that is causing it to grow. The potential for discovering mutations

in the cancer cells that could lead to a new therapeutic idea is uncertain—this is at the very frontier
of cancer research right now." Partly for that reason,
as he advised me, the cost of having it done is also
very steep at the moment. But to judge by my correspondence, practically everybody in this country
has either had cancer or has a friend or relative who
has been a victim of it. So perhaps I will be able to
contribute a little bit to enlarging the knowledge
that will help future generations.

—

I say "perhaps" partly because Francis has now had
to lay aside a lot of his pioneering work, in order
to defend his profession from a legal blockade of
its most promising avenue of endeavor. Even as he
and I were having those partly thrilling and partly
lowering conversations, last August a federal judge
in Washington, D.C., ordered a halt to all government expenditure on embryonic stem-cell research.
Judge Royce Lamberth was responding to a suit
from supporters of the so-called Dickey-Wicker
Amendment, named for the Republican duo who
in 1995 managed to forbid federal spending on any
research that employs a human embryo. As a believ-

ing Christian, Francis is squeamish about the creation for research purposes of these nonsentient cell clumps (as, if you care, am I), but he was hoping for good work to result from the use of *already existing* embryos, originally created for in vitro fertilization. These embryos are going nowhere as it is. But now religious maniacs strive to forbid even their use, which would help what the same maniacs regard as the unformed embryo's fellow humans! The politicized sponsors of this pseudo-scientific nonsense should be ashamed to live, let alone die. If you want to take part in the "war" against cancer, and other terrible maladies, too, then join the battle against their lethal stupidity.

IV

*E*VER SINCE I WAS FELLED IN MID–BOOK TOUR IN THE summer of 2010, I have adored and seized all chances to play catch-up and to keep as many engagements as I can. Debating and lecturing are part of the breath of life to me, and I take deep drafts whenever and wherever possible. I also truly enjoy the face time with you, dear reader, whether or not you bring a receipt for a shiny new copy of my memoirs. But here is what happened a few weeks ago. Picture, if you will, me sitting at my table, approached by a motherly-looking woman (a key constituent of my demographic):

SHE: I was so sorry to hear you had been ill.

ME: Thank you for saying so.

SHE: A cousin of mine had cancer.

ME: Oh, I *am* sorry to hear that.

SHE: [*As the line of customers lengthens behind her*] Yes, in his liver.

ME: That's never good.

SHE: But it went away, after the doctors had told him it was incurable.

ME: Well, that's what we all want to hear.

SHE: [*With those farther back in line now showing signs of impatience*] Yes. But then it came back, *much* worse than before.

ME: Oh, how dreadful.

SHE: And then he died. It was agonizing. *Agonizing.* Seemed to take him forever.

ME: [*Beginning to search for words*] …

SHE: Of course, he was a lifelong homosexual.

ME: [*Not quite finding the words, and not wishing to sound stupid by echoing "of course"*] …

SHE: And his whole immediate family disowned him. He died virtually alone.

ME: Well, I hardly know what to …

SHE: Anyway, I just wanted you to know that I understand *exactly* what you are going through.

This was a surprisingly exhausting encounter, without which I could easily have done. It made me wonder if perhaps there was room for a short handbook of cancer etiquette. This would apply to sufferers as well as to sympathizers. After all, I have hardly been reticent about my own malady. But nor do I walk around sporting a huge lapel button that reads, ASK ME ABOUT STAGE FOUR METASTASIZED ESOPHAGEAL CANCER, AND ONLY ABOUT THAT. In truth, if you can't bring me news about that and that alone, and about what happens when lymph nodes and lung may be involved, I am not all that interested or all that knowledgeable. One almost develops a kind of elitism about the uniqueness of one's own personal disorder. So, if your own first- or secondhand tale is about some other organs, you might want to consider telling it sparingly, or at least more selectively. This suggestion applies whether the story is intensely depressing and lowering to the spirit—see above—or whether it is intended to convey uplift and optimism: "My grandmother was diagnosed with terminal melanoma of the G-spot and they just about gave up on her. But she hung in there and took huge doses of chemotherapy and radiation at the same time, and the last postcard we had was from her at the top of Mount Everest." Once again, your narrative may fail to grip if you haven't taken any care to find out how well or badly your audience member is faring (or feeling).

It's normally agreed that the question "How are you?" doesn't put you on your oath to give a full or honest answer. So when asked these days, I tend to say something cryptic like, "A bit early to say." (If it's the wonderful staff at my oncology clinic who inquire, I sometimes go so far as to respond, "I seem to have cancer today.") Nobody wants to be told about the countless minor horrors and humiliations that become facts of "life" when your body turns from being a friend to being a foe: the boring switch from chronic constipation to its sudden dramatic opposite; the equally nasty double cross of feeling acute hunger while fearing even the scent of food; the absolute misery of gut-wringing nausea on an utterly empty stomach; or the pathetic discovery that hair loss extends to the disappearance of the follicles in your nostrils, and thus to the childish and irritating phenomenon of a permanently runny nose. Sorry, but you did ask... It's no fun to appreciate to the full the truth of the materialist proposition that I don't *have* a body, I *am* a body.

But it's not really possible to adopt a stance of "Don't ask, don't tell," either. Like its original, this is a prescription for hypocrisy and double standards. Friends and relatives, obviously, don't really have the option of not making kind inquiries. One way of trying to put them at their ease is to be as candid as possible and not to adopt any sort of euphemism or denial. The swiftest way of doing this is to note that the thing about Stage Four is that there is no such thing as Stage Five. Quite rightly, some take me up on it. I recently had to accept that I wasn't going to be able to attend my niece's wedding, in my old hometown and former university in Oxford. This depressed me for more than one reason, and an especially close friend inquired, "Is it that you're afraid you'll never see England again?" As it happens he was exactly right to ask, and it had been precisely that which had been bothering me, but I was unreasonably shocked by his bluntness. I'll do the facing of hard facts, thanks. Don't you be doing it too. And yet I had absolutely invited the question. Telling someone else, with deliberate realism, that once I'd had a few more scans and treatments I might be told by the doctors that things from now on could be mainly a matter of "management," I again had the wind knocked out of me when she said, "Yes, I suppose a time comes when you have to consider letting go." How true, and how crisp a summary of what I had just said myself. But again there was the unreasonable urge to have a kind of monopoly on, or a sort of veto over, what was actually sayable. Cancer victimhood contains a permanent temptation to be self-centered and even solipsistic.

So my proposed etiquette handbook would impose duties on me as well as upon those who say too much, or too little, in an attempt to cover the inevitable awkwardness in diplomatic relations between Tumortown and its neighbors. If you want an instance of exactly how not to be an envoy from the former, I would offer you both the book and the video of *The Last Lecture.* It would be in bad taste to say that this—a pre-recorded farewell by the late professor Randy Pausch—had "gone viral" on the Internet, but so it has. It should bear its own health warning: so sugary that you may need an insulin shot to withstand it. Pausch used to work for Disney and it shows. He includes a whole section in defense of cliché, not omitting, "Other than that, Mrs. Lincoln, how was the play?" The words "kid" or "childhood" and "dream" are employed as if for the very first time. ("Anyone who uses 'childhood' and 'dream' in the same sentence usually gets my attention.") Pausch taught at Carnegie Mellon, but it's the *Dale* Carnegie note that he likes to strike. ("Brick walls are there for a reason…to give us a chance to show how badly we want something.") Of course, you don't have to read Pausch's book, but many students and colleagues did have to attend the lecture, at which Pausch did push-ups, showed home videos, mugged for the camera, and generally joshed his head off. It ought to be an offense to be excruciating and unfunny in circumstances where your audience is almost morally obliged to enthuse. This was as much an intrusion, in its way, as that of the relentless motherly persecutor with whom I began. As the populations of Tumortown and Wellville continue to swell and to "interact," there's a growing need for ground rules that prevent us from inflicting ourselves upon one another.

V

I have seen the moment of my greatness flicker,
And I have seen the eternal Footman hold my coat, and
  snicker,
And in short, I was afraid.

> —T. S. Eliot, "The Love Song of
> J. Alfred Prufrock"

LIKE SO MANY OF LIFE'S VARIETIES OF EXPERIENCE, the novelty of a diagnosis of malignant cancer has a tendency to wear off. The thing begins to pall, even to become banal. One can become quite used to the specter of the eternal Footman, like some lethal old bore lurking in the hallway at the end of the evening, hoping for the chance to have a word. And I don't so much object to his holding my coat in that marked manner, as if mutely reminding me that it's time to be on my way. No, it's the *snickering* that gets me down.

On a much too regular basis, the disease serves me up with a teasing special of the day, or a flavor of the month. It might be random sores and ulcers, on the tongue or in the mouth. Or why not a touch of peripheral neuropathy, involving numb and chilly feet? Daily existence becomes a babyish thing, measured out not in Prufrock's coffee spoons but in tiny doses of nourishment, accompanied by heartening noises from onlookers, or solemn discussions of the operations of the digestive system, conducted with motherly strangers. On the less good days, I feel like that wooden-legged piglet belonging to a sadistically sentimental family that could bear to eat him only a chunk at a time. Except that cancer isn't so... considerate.

Most despond-inducing and alarming of all, so far, was the moment when my voice suddenly rose to a childish (or perhaps piglet-like) piping squeak. It then began to register all over the place, from a gruff and husky whisper to a papery, plaintive bleat. And at times it threatened, and now threatens daily, to disappear altogether. I had just returned from giving a couple of speeches in California, where with the help of morphine and adrenaline I could still successfully "project" my utterances, when I made an attempt to hail a taxi outside my home— and nothing happened. I stood, frozen, like a silly cat that had abruptly lost its meow. I used to be able to stop a New York cab at thirty paces. I could also, without the help of a microphone, reach the back row and gallery of a crowded debating hall. And it may be nothing to boast about, but people tell me that if their radio or television was on, even in the next room, they could always pick out my tones and know that I was "on" too.

Like health itself, the loss of such a thing can't be imagined until it occurs. In common with everybody else, I have played versions of the youthful "Which would you rather?" game, in which most usually it's debated whether blindness or deafness would be the most oppressive. But I don't ever recall speculating much about being struck dumb. (In the American vernacular, to say "I'd really hate to be dumb" might in any case draw another snicker.)

Deprivation of the ability to speak is more like an attack of impotence, or the amputation of part of the personality. To a great degree, in public and private, I "was" my voice. All the rituals and etiquette of conversation, from clearing the throat in preparation for the telling of an extremely long and taxing joke to (in younger days) trying to make my proposals more persuasive as I sank the tone by a strategic octave of shame, were innate and essential to me. I have never been able to sing, but I could once recite poetry and quote prose and was sometimes even asked to do so. And timing is everything: the exquisite moment when one can break in and cap a story, or turn a line for a laugh, or ridicule an opponent. I lived for moments like that. Now if I want to enter a conversation, I have to attract attention in some other way, and live with the awful fact that people are then listening "sympathetically." At least they don't have to pay attention for long: I can't keep it up and anyway can't stand to.

When you fall ill, people send you CDs. Very often, in my experience, these are by Leonard Cohen. So I have recently learned a song, entitled "If It Be Your

Will." It's a tiny bit saccharine, but it's beautifully rendered and it opens like this:

If it be your will,
That I speak no more,
And my voice be still,
As it was before…

I find it's best not to listen to this late at night. Leonard Cohen is unimaginable without, and indissoluble from, his voice. (I now doubt that I could be bothered, or bear, to hear that song done by anybody else.) In some ways, I tell myself, I could hobble along by communicating only in writing. But this is really only because of my age. If I had been robbed of my voice earlier, I doubt that I could ever have achieved much on the page. I owe a vast debt to Simon Hoggart of the *Guardian* (son of the author of *The Uses of Literacy*), who about thirty-five years ago informed me that an article of mine was well argued but dull, and advised me briskly to write "more like the way you talk." At the time, I was near speechless at the charge of being boring and never thanked him properly, but in time I appreciated that my fear of self-indulgence and the personal pronoun was its own form of indulgence.

To my writing classes I used later to open by saying that anybody who could talk could also write. Having cheered them up with this easy-to-grasp ladder, I then replaced it with a huge and loathsome snake: "How many people in this class, would you say, can talk? I mean really talk?" That had its duly woeful effect. I told them to read every composition aloud, preferably to a trusted friend. The rules are much the same: Avoid stock expressions (like the plague, as William Safire used to say) and repetitions. Don't say that as a boy your grandmother used to read to you, unless at that stage of her life she really *was* a boy, in which case you have probably thrown away a better intro. If something is worth hearing or listening to, it's very probably worth reading. So, this above all: Find your own *voice*.

The most satisfying compliment a reader can pay is to tell me that he or she feels personally addressed. Think of your own favorite authors and see if that isn't precisely one of the things that engages you, often at first without your noticing it. A good conversation is the only human equivalent: the realizing that decent points are being made and understood, that irony is in play, and elaboration, and that a dull or obvious remark would be almost physically hurtful. This is how philosophy evolved in the symposium, before philosophy was written down. And poetry began with the voice as its only player and the ear as its only recorder. Indeed, I don't know of any really good writer who was deaf, either. How could one ever come, even with the clever signage of the good Abbé de l'Épée, to appreciate the minuscule twinges and ecstasies of nuance that the well-tuned voice imparts? Henry James and Joseph Conrad actually *dictated* their later novels—which must count as one of the greatest vocal achievements of all time, even though they might have benefited from hearing some passages read back to them—and Saul Bellow dictated much of *Humboldt's Gift*. Without our corresponding feeling for the idiolect, the stamp on the way an individual actually talks, and therefore writes, we would be deprived of a whole continent of human sympathy, and of its minor-key pleasures such as mimicry and parody.

More solemnly: "All I have is a voice," wrote W. H. Auden in "September 1, 1939," his agonized attempt to comprehend, and oppose, the triumph of radical evil. "Who can reach the deaf?" he asked despairingly. "Who can speak for the dumb?" At about the same time, the German-Jewish future Nobelist Nelly Sachs found that the apparition of Hitler had caused her to become literally speechless: robbed of her very voice by the stark negation of all values. Our own everyday idiom preserves the idea, however mildly: When a devoted public servant dies, the obituaries will often say that he was "a voice" for the unheard.

From the human throat terrible banes can also emerge: bawling, droning, whining, yelling, inciting ("the windiest militant trash," as Auden phrased it in the same poem), and even snickering. It's the chance to pitch still, small voices against this torrent of babble and noise, the voices of wit and understatement, for which one yearns. All of the best recollections of wisdom and friendship, from Plato's "Apology" for Socrates to Boswell's *Life of Johnson*, resound with the spoken, unscripted moments of interplay and reason and speculation. It's in engagements like this, in competition and comparison with others, that one can hope to hit upon the elusive, magical *mot juste*. For me, to remember friendship is to recall those conversations that it seemed a sin to break off: the ones that made the sacrifice of the following day a trivial one. That was the way that Callimachus chose to remember his beloved Heraclitus (as adapted into English by William Cory):

They told me, Heraclitus; they told me you were dead.
They brought me bitter news to hear, and bitter tears
    to shed.
I wept when I remembered how often you and I
Had tired the sun with talking, and sent him down
    the sky.

Indeed, he rests his claim for his friend's immortality on the sweetness of his tones:

Still are thy pleasant voices, thy nightingales, awake;
For Death, he taketh all away, but them he cannot take.

Perhaps a little too much uplift in that closing line…

<hr />

In the medical literature, the vocal "cord" is a mere "fold," a piece of gristle that strives to reach out and touch its twin, thus producing the possibility of sound effects. But I feel that there must be a deep relationship with the word "chord": the resonant vibration that can stir memory, produce music, evoke love, bring tears, move crowds to pity and mobs to passion. We may not be, as we used to boast, the only animals capable of speech. But we are the only ones who can deploy vocal communication for sheer pleasure and recreation, combining it with our two other boasts of reason and humor to produce higher syntheses. To lose this ability is to be deprived of an entire range of faculty: It is assuredly to die more than a little.

My chief consolation in this year of living dyingly has been the presence of friends. I can't eat or drink for pleasure anymore, so when they offer to come it's only for the blessed chance to talk. Some of these comrades can easily fill a hall with paying customers avid to hear them: They are talkers with whom it's a privilege just to keep up. Now at least I can do the listening for free. Can they come and see me? Yes, but only in a way. So now every day I go to a waiting room, and watch the awful news from Japan on cable TV (often closed-captioned, just to torture myself) and wait impatiently for a high dose of protons to be fired into my body at two-thirds the speed of light. What do I hope for? If not a cure, then a remission. And what do I want back? In the most beautiful apposition of two of the simplest words in our language: the freedom of speech.

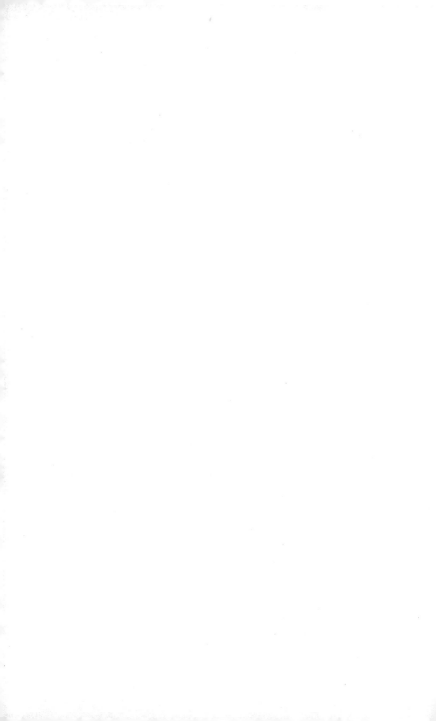

VI

Death has this much to be said for it:
You don't have to get out of bed for it.
Wherever you happen to be
They bring it to you—free.

—Kingsley Amis

Pointed threats, they bluff with scorn
Suicide remarks are torn
From the fool's gold mouthpiece the hollow horn
Plays wasted words, proves to warn
That he not busy being born is busy dying.

—Bob Dylan, "It's Alright, Ma
(I'm Only Bleeding)"

W HEN IT CAME TO IT, AND OLD KINGSLEY SUFFERED from a demoralizing and disorienting fall, he did take to his bed and eventually turned his face to the wall. It wasn't all reclining and waiting for hospital room service after that—"Kill me, you fucking fool!" he once alarmingly exclaimed to his son Philip—but essentially he waited passively for the end. It duly came, without much fuss and with no charge.

Mr. Robert Zimmerman of Hibbing, Minnesota, has had at least one very close encounter with death, more than one update and revision of his relationship with the almighty and the Four Last Things, and looks set to go on demonstrating that there are many different ways of proving that one is alive. After all, considering the alternatives…

Before I was diagnosed with esophageal cancer a year and a half ago, I rather jauntily told the readers of my memoirs that when faced with extinction I wanted to be fully conscious and awake, in order to "do" death in the active and not the passive sense. And I do, still, try to nurture that little flame of curiosity and defiance: willing to play out the string to the end and wishing to be spared nothing that properly belongs to a life span. However, one thing that grave illness does is to make you examine familiar principles and seemingly reliable sayings. And there's one that I find I am not saying with quite the same conviction as I once used to: In particular, I have slightly stopped issuing the announcement that "whatever doesn't kill me makes me stronger."

In fact, I now sometimes wonder why I ever thought it profound. It is usually attributed to Friedrich Nietzsche: *Was mich nicht umbringt macht mich stärker.* In German it reads and sounds more like poetry, which is why it seems probable to me that Nietzsche borrowed it from Goethe, who was writing a century earlier. But does the rhyme suggest a reason? Perhaps it does, or can, in matters of the emotions. I can remember thinking, of testing moments involving love and hate, that I had, so to speak, come out of them ahead, with some strength accrued from the experience that I couldn't have acquired any other way. And then once or twice, walking away from a car wreck or a close encounter with mayhem while doing foreign reporting, I experienced a rather fatuous feeling of having been toughened by the encounter. But really, that's to say no more than "There but for the grace of god go I," which in turn is to say no more than "The grace of god has happily embraced me and skipped that unfortunate other man."

～

In the brute physical world, and the one encompassed by medicine, there are all too many things that could kill you, don't kill you, and then leave you considerably weaker. Nietzsche was destined to find this out in the hardest possible way, which makes it additionally perplexing that he chose to include the maxim in his 1889 anthology *Twilight of the Idols*. (In German this is rendered as *Götzen-Dämmerung*, which contains a clear echo of Wagner's epic. Possibly his great quarrel with the composer, in which he recoiled with horror from Wagner's repudiation of the classics in favor of German blood myths and legends, was one of the things that did lend Nietzsche moral strength and fortitude. Certainly the book's subtitle—"How to Philosophize with a Hammer"— has plenty of bravado.)

In the remainder of his life, however, Nietzsche seems to have caught an early dose of syphilis, very probably during his first ever sexual encounter, which gave him crushing migraine headaches and attacks of blindness and metastasized into dementia and paralysis. This, while it did not kill him right away, certainly contributed to his death and cannot possibly, in the meanwhile, be said to have made him stronger. In the course of his mental decline, he became convinced that the most important possible cultural feat would be to prove that the plays of Shakespeare had been written by Bacon. This is an unfailing sign of advanced intellectual and mental prostration.

(I take a slight interest in this, because not long ago I was invited onto a Christian radio station in deepest Dixie to debate religion. My interviewer maintained a careful southern courtesy throughout, always allowing me enough time to make my points, and then surprised me by inquiring if I regarded myself as in any sense a Nietzschean. I replied in the negative, saying that I had agreed with some arguments put forward by the great man but didn't owe any large insight to him and found his contempt for democracy to be somewhat off-putting. H. L. Mencken and others, I tried to add, had also used him to argue some crude social-Darwinist points about the pointlessness of aiding the "unfit." And his frightful sister, Elisabeth, had exploited his decline to misuse his work as if it had been written in support of the German anti-Semitic nationalist movement. This had perhaps given Nietzsche an undeserved posthumous reputation as a fanatic. The questioner pressed on, asking if I knew that much of Nietzsche's work had been produced while he was decaying from terminal syphilis. I again responded that I had heard this and knew of no reason to doubt it, though I knew of no confirmation either. Just as it became too late, and I heard the strains of music and the words that this would be all we would have time for, my host stole a march and wondered how much of my own writing on god had perhaps been influenced by a similar malady! I should have seen this "gotcha" coming, but was left wordless.)

Eventually, and in miserable circumstances in the Italian city of Turin, Nietzsche was overwhelmed at the sight of a horse being cruelly beaten in the street. Rushing to throw his arms around the animal's neck, he suffered some terrible seizure and seems for the rest of his pain-racked and haunted life to have been under the care of his mother and sister. The date of the Turin trauma is potentially interesting. It occurred in 1889, and we know that in 1887 Nietzsche had been powerfully influenced by his discovery of the works of Dostoyevsky. There appears to be an almost eerie correspondence between the episode in the street and the awful graphic dream experienced by Raskolnikov on the night before he commits the decisive murders in *Crime and Punishment.* The nightmare, which is quite impossible to forget once you have read it, involves the terribly prolonged beating to death of a horse. Its owner scourges it across the eyes, smashes its spine with a pole, calls on bystanders to help with the flogging...we are spared nothing. If the gruesome coincidence was enough to bring about Nietzsche's final unhingment, then he must have been tremendously weakened, or made appallingly vulnerable, by his other, unrelated sufferings. These, then, by no means served to make him stronger. The most he could have meant, I now think, is that he made the most of his few intervals from pain and madness to set down his collections of penetrating aphorism and paradox. This may have given him the euphoric impression that he was triumphing, and making use of the Will to Power. *Twilight of the Idols* was actually published almost simultaneously with the horror in Turin, so the coincidence was pushed as far as it could reasonably go.

Or take an example from an altogether different and more temperate philosopher, nearer to our own time. The late Professor Sidney Hook was a famous materialist and pragmatist, who wrote sophisticated treatises that synthesized the work of John Dewey and Karl Marx. He, too, was an unrelenting atheist. Toward the end of his long life he became seriously ill and began to reflect on the paradox that—based as he was in the medical mecca of Stanford, California—he was able to avail himself of a historically unprecedented level of care, while at the same time being exposed to a degree of suffering that previous generations might not have been able to afford. Reasoning on this after one especially horrible experience from which he had eventually recovered, he decided that he would after all rather have died:

> I lay at the point of death. A congestive heart failure was treated for diagnostic purposes by an angiogram that triggered a stroke. Violent and painful hiccups, uninterrupted for several days and nights, prevented the ingestion of

food. My left side and one of my vocal cords became paralyzed. Some form of pleurisy set in, and I felt I was drowning in a sea of slime. In one of my lucid intervals during those days of agony, I asked my physician to discontinue all life-supporting services or show me how to do it.

The physician denied this plea, rather loftily assuring Hook that "someday I would appreciate the unwisdom of my request." But the stoic philosopher, from the vantage point of continued life, still insisted that he wished he had been permitted to expire. He gave three reasons. Another agonizing stroke could hit him, forcing him to suffer it all over again. His family was being put through a hellish experience. Medical resources were being pointlessly expended. In the course of his essay, he used a potent phrase to describe the position of others who suffer like this, referring to them as lying on "mattress graves."

If being restored to life doesn't count as something that doesn't kill you, then what does? And yet there seems no meaningful sense in which it made Sidney Hook "stronger." Indeed, if anything, it seems to have concentrated his attention on the way in which each debilitation builds on its predecessor and becomes one cumulative misery with only one possible outcome. After all, if it were otherwise, then each attack, each stroke, each vile hiccup, each slime assault, would collectively build one up and strengthen resistance. And this is plainly absurd. So we are left with something quite unusual in the annals of unsentimental approaches to extinction: not the wish to die with dignity but the desire *to have died*.

—————

Professor Hook eventually left us in 1989, and I am a generation younger than him. I haven't sailed as close to the bitter end as he had to do. Nor have I yet had to think of having such an arduous conversation with a physician. But I do remember lying there and looking down at my naked torso, which was covered almost from throat to navel by a vivid red radiation rash. This was the product of a monthlong bombardment with protons which had burned away all of the cancer in my clavicular and paratracheal nodes, as well as the original tumor in the esophagus. This put me in a rare class of patients who could claim to have received the highly advanced expertise uniquely available at the stellar zip code of MD Anderson Cancer Center in Houston. To say the rash hurt would be pointless. The struggle is to convey the way that it hurt *on the inside.* I lay for days on end, trying in vain to postpone the moment when I would have to swallow. Every time I did swallow, a hellish tide of pain would flow up my throat, culminating in what felt like a mule kick in the small of my back. I wondered if things looked as red and inflamed within as they did without. And then I had an unprompted rogue thought: If I had been told about all this in advance, would I have opted for the treatment? There were several moments as I bucked and writhed and gasped and cursed when I seriously doubted it.

It's probably a merciful thing that pain is impossible to describe from memory. It's also impossible to warn against. If my proton doctors had tried to tell me up front, they might perhaps have spoken of "grave discomfort" or perhaps of a burning sensation. I only know that nothing at all could have readied or steadied me for this thing that seemed to scorn painkillers and to attack me in my core. I now seem to have run out of radiation options in those spots (thirty-five straight days being considered as much as anyone can take), and while this isn't in any way good news, it spares me from having to wonder if I could willingly endure the same course of treatment again.

But mercifully, too, I now can't summon the memory of how I felt during those lacerating days and nights. And I've since had some intervals of relative robustness. So as a rational actor, taking the radiation together with the reaction and the recovery, I have to agree that if I had declined the first stage, thus avoiding the second and the third, I would already be dead. And this has no appeal.

However, there is no escaping the fact that I am otherwise enormously weaker than I was then. How long ago it seems that I presented the proton team with champagne and then hopped almost nimbly into a taxi. During my next hospital stay, in Washington, D.C., the institution gifted me with a vicious staph pneumonia (and sent me home twice with it) that almost snuffed me out. The annihilating fatigue that came over me in consequence also contained the deadly threat of surrender to the inescapable: I would often find fatalism and resignation washing drearily over me as I failed to battle my general inanition. Only two things rescued me from betraying myself and letting go: a wife who would not hear of me talking in this boring and useless way, and various friends who also spoke freely. Oh, and the regular painkiller. How happily I measured off my day as I saw the injection being readied. It counted as a real event. With some analgesics, if you are lucky, you can actually feel the hit as it goes in: a sort of warming tingle with an idiotic bliss to it. To have come to this—like the sad goons who raid pharmacies for OxyContin. But it was an alleviation of boredom, and a guilty pleasure (not many of those in Tumortown), and not least a relief from pain.

In my English family, the role of national poet was taken not by Philip Larkin but by John Betjeman, bard of suburbia and the middle class and a much more mordant presence than the rather teddy-bearish figure he sometimes presented to the world. His poem "Five O'Clock Shadow" shows him at his least furry:

This is the time of day when we in the Men's Ward
Think "One more surge of the pain and I give up the
 fight,"
When he who struggles for breath can struggle less
 strongly:
This is the time of day that is worse than night.

I have come to know that feeling all right: the sensation and conviction that the pain will never go away and that the wait for the next fix is unjustly long. Then a sudden fit of breathlessness, followed by some pointless coughing and then—if it's a lousy day—by more expectoration than I can handle. Pints of old saliva, occasionally mucus, and what the hell do I need *heartburn* for at this exact moment? It's not as if I have eaten anything: a tube delivers all my nourishment. All of this, and the childish resentment that goes with it, constitutes a weakening. So does the amazing weight loss that the tube seems unable to combat. I have now lost almost a third of my body mass since the cancer was diagnosed: It may not kill me, but the atrophy of muscle makes it harder to take even the simple exercises without which I'll become more enfeebled still.

—≈—

I am typing this having just had an injection to try to reduce the pain in my arms, hands, and fingers. The chief side effect of this pain is numbness in the extremities, filling me with the not irrational fear that I shall lose the ability to write. Without that ability, I feel sure in advance, my "will to live" would be hugely attenuated. I often grandly say that writing is not just my living and my livelihood but my very life, and it's true. Almost like the threatened loss of my voice, which is currently being alleviated by some temporary injections into my vocal folds, I feel my personality and identity dissolving as I contemplate dead hands and the loss of the transmission belts that connect me to writing and thinking.

These are progressive weaknesses that in a more "normal" life might have taken decades to catch up with me. But, as with the normal life, one finds that every passing day represents more and more relentlessly subtracted from less and less. In other words, the process both etiolates you and moves you nearer toward death. How could it be otherwise? Just as I was beginning to reflect along these lines, I came across an article on the treatment of post-traumatic stress disorder. We now know, from dearly bought experience, much more about this malady than we used to. Apparently, one of the symptoms by which it is made known is that a tough veteran will say, seeking to make light of his experience, that "what didn't kill me made me stronger." This is one of the manifestations that "denial" takes.

I am attracted to the German etymology of the

word "stark," and its relative used by Nietzsche, *stärker*, which means "stronger." In Yiddish, to call someone a *shtarker* is to credit him with being a militant, a tough guy, a hard worker. So far, I have decided to take whatever my disease can throw at me, and to stay combative even while taking the measure of my inevitable decline. I repeat, this is no more than what a healthy person has to do in slower motion. It is our common fate. In either case, though, one can dispense with facile maxims that don't live up to their apparent billing.

I may have made one exception to my emerging rule that Nietzsche was to be distrusted, or to my pretense to myself that I had resources that I may not have truly possessed. A good deal of cancer life has to do with the blood, of which cancer is indeed the particular malady. A sufferer will find himself "giving" quite a quantity of the fluid, either to facilitate the opening of a catheter or to help test the levels of blood sugar and other material. For years, I found it absurdly easy to undergo routine blood tests. I would walk in, sit down, endure a brief squeeze from a tourniquet until a usable vein became available or accessible, and then a single small stab would allow the filling of the relevant little tubes and syringes.

Over time, however, this ceased to be one of the pleasurable highlights of the medicalized day. The phlebotomist would sit down, take my hand or wrist in his or her hand, and sigh. The welts of reddish and purple could already be seen, giving the arm a definite "junkie" look. The veins themselves lay sunken in their beds, either hollow or crushed. Very occasionally, they would cooperate with a junkie-based strategy that consisted of slowly smacking them with taut fingertips, but this seldom yielded a robust result. Large swellings would occur, usually just near the elbow or wrist joint, or anywhere they would do the least good.

In addition, one had to stop pretending that the business was effectively painless. No more the jaunty talk of "one little pinch." It doesn't actually hurt *that much* to have a probing needle inserted for a second time. No, what hurts is having it moved to and fro, in the hope that it can properly penetrate the vein and release the needful fluid. And the more this is done, the more it hurts. This illustrates the whole business in microcosm: the "battle" against cancer reduced to a struggle to get a few drops of gore out of a large warm mammal that cannot provide them. Please believe me when I say that one quickly comes to sympathize with the technicians. They are proud of their work, and do not enjoy imposing "discomfort." Indeed, they will regularly and with relief give place to another volunteer or submit to another's expertise.

But the job has to be done, and there is dismay when it can't be completed. I was recently scheduled for the insertion of a "PIC" line, by means of which a permanent blood catheter is inserted in the upper arm, so that the need for repeated temporary invasions can be obviated. The experts told me that this seldom took more than ten minutes to complete (which had been my own experience on previous visits). It can't have been much less than two hours until, having tried and failed with both arms, I was lying between two bed-pads that were liberally laced with dried or clotting blood. The upset of the nurses was palpable. And we were further off from a solution.

As this kind of thing became more common, I began to take on the role of morale-booster. When the technician would offer to stop, I would urge her to go on and assure her that I sympathized. I would relate the number of attempts made on previous occasions, in order to spur greater efforts. My self-image was that of the plucky English immigrant, rising above the agony of a little needle-stick. Whatever didn't kill me, I averred, would make me stronger…I think this began to pall on the day that I had asked to "keep going" through eleven sessions, and was secretly hoping for the chance to give up and go to sleep. Then suddenly the worried face of the expert cleared all at once as he exclaimed, "Well, twelve times is the charm," and the life-giving thread began to unspool in the syringe. From this time on, it seemed absurd to affect the idea that this bluffing on my part was making me stronger, or making other people perform more strongly or cheerfully either. Whatever view one takes of the outcome being affected by morale, it seems certain that the realm of illusion must be escaped before anything else.

VII

NOT MANY WEEKS AGO, I WAS STARTING A BEDridden day in a state of acute powerlessness and quite rough pain. As I lay unable to move but braced from past experience, I heard a soothing and capable voice saying, "Now you might feel just a little prick." (Be assured: Male patients have exhausted all the possibilities of this feeble joke within the first few days of hearing it.) And almost at once I felt reassured in a different way, because that voice and that expression and that little pang meant that the pain would lift and my limbs straighten, and my day begin. And so it proved.

What if, though, as I once semi-consciously

thought as I lay in similar distress, that friendly voice had had just the faintest hint of a taunt in it? What if it had been saying, in the merest possible way, "This won't hurt—*much*"? The whole balance of power would have been violently subverted, leaving me defenseless and petrified. I would also, instantly, have to wonder how long I could coexist with such a threat. The torturer's intricate work would have begun.

I stress "intricate" because torture isn't really a matter of sheer brute pain and force. As I found out when I was actually a torture victim, it is above all a matter of subtle calibration. "How are we *doing* today? Any *discomfort*?" This is made additionally problematic by the tendency of modern medicine to fall back on the use of euphemistic words in any case, the polite evasion of the weak "discomfort" being one of the most salient of these. Another avenue of euphemism is laid out by the planned and coordinated approach; thus one might hear the question, "Have you met with our 'pain management' team yet?" Once you have heard it the wrong way, this can seem like an echo of the torturer's practice, of showing to the victim the instruments that will be used upon him, or describing the range of techniques, and letting these threats do the main part of the job. (Galileo Galilei was allegedly exposed to this while undergoing the graduated pressure that eventually squeezed him to recant.)

I became a torture victim because I wanted the readers of *Vanity Fair* to have an idea of what was involved in the sordid and obscure controversy about "waterboarding." And the only way left, or left untried, was to offer myself to this "procedure." Obviously there were limits to the authenticity of its infliction—and I had to be in some sense "in control" of the setting—but I was determined as far as possible to discover what a "waterboarded" person really undergoes. With the help of some very serious former Special Forces personnel, who knew that they were breaking American law on American soil, I arranged an appointment in the hills of North Carolina. Before we could even begin, I had signed a legal document indemnifying them in case they killed me by the infliction of physical or psychological trauma (a stronger word, there).

What happens, you may have been told, is a "simulation" of the sensation of drowning. Wrong. What happens is that you are slowly but inexorably drowned. And if at any point you manage to evade the deadly drip of water, your torturer will know. He or she will then make a minute but effective adjustment. When I interviewed my torturers later I was particularly interested in this aspect of matters. Oh yes, they said with mild bragging, we have lots of little moves and shakes and twists that will get the job done and not leave a mark. Again, you note this pride in technique and its almost humanist tone of professional expression. The language of torturers…

The reason I have decided to write about this in the present context is as follows. Ever since I composed and published the original essay, which was some time before I was diagnosed with esophageal cancer, I had been suffering from some form of post-torture stress that probably has yet to be classified or named. In my own case at any rate, it has to do with asphyxiation. And the "aspiration" of moisture can trigger a flood of panic and has become imbricated with the larger and deadlier symptoms of my various pneumonias. And every day, I am forced to prepare myself to be tube-fed through an apparatus of liquid nourishment, or to be washed to different degrees of immersion, or to be otherwise made highly vulnerable. So I am very fortunate indeed that I have never had to hear the torturer's odious whisper, or to shrink at the thought that I am only a wrinkle or a twist away from severe fear and "distress" (a word quite high on the euphemism scale). But I do now know how the trick could be pulled.

I have been cycled through various great American hospitals in the course of my experience, at least one of which is famous for being operated by a historic religious order. In each of the rooms of this hospital, from no matter what perspective you lie in bed, the commanding view is decidedly that of a large black metal crucifix embedded tenaciously in the wall. I had no special objection to this on one level, because it really did little more than repeat the name of the hospital itself. (I tend not to pick my fights with the chaplains' departments until I have a proper point to make. In Texas, for instance, in a purpose-built brand-new facility that took the towers to the level of more than two dozen, I got them to agree in principle that it was slightly idiotic not to boast of a thirteenth floor but instead to skip from twelve to fourteen. Surely nobody checks in here to complain of cosmic fears generated by a number, or would check out because of it: We seem incidentally quite unable to discern how this dank little superstition ever got started.)

However, I also happen to know that it was a

practice, during the wars of religion and the campaigns of the Inquisition, to subject the condemned to a compulsory view of the cross until they had died. In some of the fervent paintings of the grand *autos-da-fé*, or "acts of faith," not I think excluding some of the burnings alive captured by Goya on the Plaza Mayor, we see the flame and the smoke arising from the vicinity of the victim, and then the cross itself held grimly aloft before his closing eyes. I have to say that, even if this is now done only in a more "palliative" fashion, it makes me feel disapproving on the grounds of its earlier sadomasochistic associations. There are banal, quotidian hospital and medical practices that remind people of state-sponsored torture. In my own case, there are also practices that I can't separate from the hell of earlier ones. Even the thought of some misapplications of water or gas, such as a moisturized or "nebulized" breathing-treatment kit, can be more than enough to make me feel critically ill. When I was first thinking of a possible title for this book, I considered annexing the line "Obscene as cancer," from Wilfred Owen's terrifying poem about death on the Western Front, "Dulce et Decorum Est." The action describes the reaction of a group of exhausted British stragglers, caught in the open during a gas attack for which they are ill-prepared:

Gas! GAS! Quick, boys!—An ecstasy of fumbling,
Fitting the clumsy helmets just in time;
But someone still was yelling out and stumbling,
And flound'ring like a man in fire or lime…
Dim, through the misty panes and thick green light,
As under a green sea, I saw him drowning.

In all my dreams, before my helpless sight,
He plunges at me, guttering, choking, drowning.

If in some smothering dreams you too could pace
Behind the wagon that we flung him in,
And watch the white eyes writhing in his face,
His hanging face, like a devil's sick of sin;
If you could hear, at every jolt, the blood
Come gargling from the froth-corrupted lungs,
Obscene as cancer, bitter as the cud
Of vile incurable sores on innocent tongues,—
My friend, you would not tell with such high zest
To children ardent for some desperate glory,
The old Lie: Dulce et decorum est
Pro patria mori.

When I, too, am sometimes forced into premature awareness by a smothering or choked nightmare sensation, I realize how essential it is that the frontiers of medicine be so tightly and punctiliously patrolled. I appreciate that within the profession itself there be not the least concession to any relaxation of that standard. The operators of that famous hospital should be ashamed of the historic role played by their order in the appalling legalization and application of torture, and I have the same right if not duty to be equally ashamed of the official policy of torture adopted by a government whose citizenship papers I had only recently taken out.

VIII

REMEMBER, YOU TOO ARE MORTAL"—HIT ME AT THE
top of my form and just as things were beginning to
plateau. My two assets my pen and my voice—and
it had to be the esophagus. All along, while burning
the candle at both ends, I'd been "straying into the
arena of the unwell" and now "a vulgar little tumor"
was evident. This alien can't want anything; if it kills
me it dies but it seems very single-minded and set in
its purpose. No real irony here, though. Must take
absolute care not to be self-pitying or self-centered.

Publisher's note: These fragmentary jottings were left unfinished at
the time of the author's death.

Always prided myself on my reasoning faculty and my stoic materialism. I don't *have* a body, I *am* a body. Yet consciously and regularly acted as if this was not true, or as if an exception would be made in my case. Feeling husky and tired on tour? See the doctor when it's over!

Lost fourteen pounds without trying. Thin at last. But don't feel lighter because walking to the fridge is like a forced march. Then again, the vicious psoriasis/excema pustules that no doctor could treat have gone, too. This must be some impressive toxin I'm taking. And a mercy for sleep purposes...but all the sleep-aids and blissful dozes seem somehow a waste of life—there's plenty of future time in which to be unconscious.

The nice men with the oxygen and the gurney and the ambulance very gently deporting me across the frontier of the well, in another country.

The alien was burrowing into me even as I wrote the jaunty words about my own prematurely announced death.

Now so many tributes that it also seems that rumors of my LIFE have also been greatly exaggerated. Lived to see most of what's going to be written about me: this too is exhilarating but hits diminishing returns when I realize how soon it, too, will be "background."

Julian Barnes on John Diamond...

A bout de soufflé...Seberg/Belmondo. Funny how one uses "breathless" or "out of breath" so casually. At Logan [airport]—can't breathe! Next stop terminal.

Tragedy? Wrong word: Hegel versus the Greeks.

Morning of biopsy, wake and say whatever happens this is the last day of my old life. No pretense of youth or youthfulness anymore. From now on an arduous awareness.

New Yorker cartoon on obit pages...Used to notice death-dates of Orwell, Wilde etc. Now maybe as long as Evelyn Waugh.

Amazing how heart and lungs and liver have held up: would have been healthier if I'd been more sickly.

PRAYER: Interesting contradictions at the expense of those who offer it—too easy a Pascalian escape-hatch with me on the right side of the wager this time: what god could ignore such supplications? Same token—those who say I am being punished are saying that god can't think of anything more vengeful than cancer for a heavy smoker.

Nose-hairs gone: runny nostrils. Constipation and diarrhea alternating...
  "The old order changeth, yielding place to new, and God fulfills himself in many ways and soon, I suppose, I shall be swept away by some vulgar little tumor..."

Some years ago, a British journalist, John Diamond, was diagnosed with cancer, and turned his condition into a weekly column. Rightly, he maintained the same perky tone that characterized the rest of his work: rightly, he admitted cowardice and panic alongside curiosity and occasional courage. His account sounded completely authentic: this was what living with cancer entailed; nor did being ill make you a different person, or stop you having rows with your wife. Like many other readers, I used to quietly urge him on from week to week. But after a year and more…well, a certain narrative expectation inevitably built up. Hey, miracle cure! Hey, I was just having you on! No, neither of those could work as endings. Diamond had to die; and he duly, correctly (in narrative terms) did. Though—how can I put this?—a stern literary critic might complain that his story lacked compactness toward the end…

Tendency of some commiserations to sound unintentionally final, either by past tense or some other giveaway of a valedictory sort. Sending flowers not as nice as it might seem.

I'm not fighting or battling cancer—it's fighting me.

Brave? Hah! Save it for a fight you can't run away from.

Saul Bellow: Death is the dark backing that a mirror needs if we are able to see anything.

Vertiginous feeling of being kicked forward in time: catapulted toward the finish line. Trying not to think with my tumor, which would not be thinking at all. People try to make it sound as if it were an EPISODE in one's life.

ONCOLOGY/ONTOLOGY: Under the old religious dispensation, heaven would simply sentence you to be lavishly tortured and *then* executed. Montaigne: "Religion's surest foundation is the contempt for life."

Fear leads to superstition—"The Big C," though, seems mercifully to have dumped—and I'm glad nobody wants to slaughter any endangered species on my behalf.

Only OK if I say something objective and stoical: Ian remarking that a time might come when I'd have to let go: Carol asking about Rebecca's wedding "Are you afraid you won't see England again?"

Also, ordinary expressions like "expiration date"… will I outlive my Amex? My driver's license? People say—I'm in town on Friday: will you be around? WHAT A QUESTION!

COLD FEET (so far only at night): "peripheral neuropathy" is another of those words like "necrotic" that describe death-in-life of the system.

AND you lose weight but cancer isn't interested in eating your flab. It wants your muscle. The Tumortown Diet ain't much help.

Worst of all is "chemo-brain." Dull, stuporous. What if the protracted, lavish torture is only the prelude to a gruesome execution.

Body turns from reliable friend to more neutral to treacherous foe…Proust?

If I convert it's because it's better that a believer dies than that an atheist does.

Not even a race for a cure…

Paperwork the curse of Tumortown.

Misery of seeing oneself on old videos or You-Tubes…

"Gradual disclosure" not yet a problem for me.

Michael Korda's book *Man to Man*...

You can get so habituated to bad news that good news is like Breytenbach and the cake. Consolations of saying, well at least now I won't have to do THAT.

Larkin good on fear in "Aubade," with implied reproof to Hume and Lucretius for their stoicism. Fair enough in one way: atheists ought not to be offering consolation either.

Banality of cancer. Entire pest-house of side-effects. Special of the day.

See Szymborska's poem on torture and the body as a reservoir of pain.

From Alan Lightman's intricate 1993 novel *Einstein's Dreams*; set in Berne in 1905:

> With infinite life comes an infinite list of relatives. Grandparents never die, nor do great-

grandparents, great-aunts…and so on, back through the generations, all alive and offering advice. Sons never escape from the shadows of their fathers. Nor do daughters of their mothers. *No one ever comes into his own…* Such is the cost of immortality. No person is whole. No person is free.

Onstage, my husband was an impossible act to follow.

If you ever saw him at the podium, you may not share Richard Dawkins's assessment that "he was the greatest orator of our time," but you will know what I mean—or at least you won't think, *She would say that, she's his wife.*

Offstage, my husband was an impossible act to follow.

At home at one of the raucous, joyous, impromptu eight-hour dinners we often found ourselves hosting, where the table was so crammed with ambassadors, hacks, political dissidents, college students, and children that elbows were colliding and it was hard to find the space to put down a glass of wine, my husband would rise to give a toast that could go on for a stirring, spellbinding, hysterically funny twenty minutes of poetry and limerick reciting, a call to arms for a cause, and jokes. "How good it is to be us," he would say in his perfect voice.

My husband is an impossible act to follow.

And yet, now I must follow him. I have been forced to have the last word.

It was the sort of early summer evening in New York when all you can think of is living. It was June 8, 2010, to be exact, the first day of his American book tour. I ran as fast as I could down East 93rd Street, suffused with joy and excitement at the sight of him in his white suit. He was dazzling. He was also dying, though we didn't know it yet. And we wouldn't know it for certain until the day of his death.

Earlier that day he had taken a detour from his book launch to a hospital because he thought he was having a heart attack. By the time I saw him standing at the stage entrance of the 92nd Street Y that evening, he and I—and we alone—knew he might have cancer. We embraced in a shadow that only we saw and chose to defy. We were euphoric. He lifted me up and we laughed.

We went into the theater, where he conquered

yet another audience. We managed to get through a jubilant dinner in his honor and set out on a stroll back to our hotel through the perfect Manhattan night, walking more than fifty blocks. Everything was as it should be, except that it wasn't. We were living in two worlds. The old one, which never seemed more beautiful, had not yet vanished; and the new one, about which we knew little except to fear it, had not yet arrived.

The new world lasted nineteen months. During this time of what he called "living dyingly," he insisted ferociously on living, and his constitution, physical and philosophical, did all it could to stay alive.

Christopher was aiming to be among the 5 to 20 percent of those who could be cured (the odds depended on what doctor we talked to and how they interpreted the scans). Without ever deceiving himself about his medical condition, and without ever allowing me to entertain illusions about his prospects for survival, he responded to every bit of clinical and statistical good news with a radical, childlike hope. His will to keep his existence intact, to remain engaged with his preternatural intensity, was spectacular.

Thanksgiving was his favorite holiday, and I watched with awe as he organized, even as he was sick from the effects of the chemotherapy, a grand family gathering in Toronto with all his children and his father-in-law on the eve of an important debate with Tony Blair about religion. This was an occasion orchestrated by a man who told me in the hotel suite that night that this would probably be his last Thanksgiving.

Not long before, back in Washington, on a bright and balmy Indian-summer afternoon, he excitedly summoned his family and visiting friends on an outing to see the Origins of Man exhibition at the Museum of Natural History, where I watched him sprint out of a cab and up the granite steps to throw up in a trash can before leading his charges through the galleries and exuberantly impressing us with the attainments of science and reason.

Christopher's charisma never left him, not in any realm: not in public, not in private, not even in the hospital. He made a party of it, transforming the sterile, chilly, neon-lighted, humming and beeping and blinking room into a study and a salon. His artful conversation never ceased.

The constant interruptions: The poking and

prodding, the sample taking, the breathing treatments, the IV bags being changed—nothing kept him from holding court, making a point or an argument or hitting a punchline for his "guests." He listened and drew us out, and had us all laughing. He was always asking for and commenting on another newspaper, another magazine, another novel, another review copy. We stood around his bed and reclined on plastic upholstered chairs as he made us into participants in his Socratic discourses.

One night he was coughing up blood and was wheeled into the ICU for a hastily scheduled bronchoscopy. I alternated between watching over him and sleeping in a convertible chair. We lay side by side in our single beds. At one point we both woke up and started burbling like children at a sleepover party. At the time, this was the best it was going to get.

When he came to following the bronchoscopy, after the doctor told him the trouble in his windpipe was not cancer but rather pneumonia, he was still intubated but avidly scribbling notes and questions about every conceivable subject. I saved the pages of paper on which he wrote his side of the conversation. There are sweet-nothings and a picture he drew on the top of the first page and then:

Pneumonia? What type?
Am I cancer free?
Pain is hard to remember, right now, 4 to 5.
He asked after the children, and my father.
How's Edwin? Tell him I asked.
I worry about him
'Cos I love him.
I want to hear him.

Slightly down the page he wrote what he wanted me to bring him from our guesthouse in Houston:

Nietzsche, Mencken and Chesterton books. Plus all random bits paper…Maybe in one hold-all bag. Look in the drawers! Bedside, etc. Up and downstairs.

That night a dear family friend arrived from New York and was in the room when, in one of his nocturnal interludes of wakefulness and energy Christopher flashed an open, wide smile around the tube still running down his throat and wrote on his clipboard:

I'm staying here [in Houston] *until I'm cured. And then I'm taking our families on a vacation to Bermuda.*

The next morning, after they took the tube out, I came into his room to find him smiling his foxlike grin at me.

"Happy anniversary!" he called out.

A nurse came in with a small white cake, paper plates and plastic forks....

Another wedding anniversary: We are reading the newspaper on the terrace in our suite in a New York hotel. It is a faultless fall day. Our two-year-old daughter is sitting contentedly beside us, drinking a bottle. She climbs off her chair and squats down, inspecting something on the ground. She pulls the bottle out of her mouth, calls to me and points to a large, motionless bumble bee. She is alarmed, shaking her head back and forth, as if to say "No, no, no!"

"The bee stopped," she says. Then she makes a command: "Make it start."

Back then she believed I had the power to reanimate the dead. I don't recall what I said to her about the bee. What I do recall are the words "Make it start." Christopher then lifted her into his lap and consoled and distracted her with a change of subject and humor. Just as he would, with all of his children, so many years later, when he was ill.

I miss his perfect voice. I heard it day and night, night and day. I miss the first happy trills when he woke; the low octaves of "his morning voice" as he read me snippets from the newspaper that outraged or amused him; the delighted and irritated (mostly irritated) registers as I interrupted him while he read; the jazz-tone riffs of him "talking down the line" to a radio station from the kitchen phone as he cooked lunch; his chirping, high-note greeting when our daughter came home from school; and his last soothing, pianissimo chatterings on retiring late at night.

I miss, as his readers must, his writer's voice, his voice on the page. I miss the unpublished Hitch: the countless notes he left for me in the entryway, on my pillow, the emails he would send while we sat in different rooms in our apartment or in our place in California and the emails he sent when he was on the road. And I miss his handwritten communiqués: his innumerable letters and postcards (we date back to the time of the epistle) and his faxes, the thrill of receiving Christopher's instant dispatches as he checked-in from a dicey spot on some other continent.

The first time Christopher went public and wrote about his illness for *Vanity Fair*, he was ambivalent about it. He was intent on protecting our family's privacy. He was living the topic and he didn't want it to become all-encompassing, he didn't want to be defined by it. He wanted to think and write in a sphere apart from sickness. He had made a pact with his editor and chum, Graydon Carter, that he would write about anything except sports, and he kept that promise. He had often put himself in the frame, but now he was the ultimate subject of the story.

His last words of the unfinished fragmentary jottings at the end of this little book may seem to trail off, but in fact they were written on his computer in bursts of energy and enthusiasm as he sat in the hospital using his food tray for a desk.

When he was admitted to the hospital for the last time, we thought it would be for a brief stay. He thought—we all thought—he'd have the chance to write the longer book that was forming in his mind. His intellectual curiosity was sparked by genomics and the cutting-edge proton radiation treatments he underwent, and he was encouraged by the prospect that his case could contribute to future medical breakthroughs. He told an editor friend waiting for an article, "Sorry for the delay, I'll be back home soon." He told me he couldn't wait to catch up on all the movies he had missed and to see the King Tut exhibition in Houston, our temporary residence.

The end was unexpected.

At home in Washington, I pull books off the shelves, out of the book towers on the floor, off the stacks of volumes on tables. Inside the back covers are notes written in his hand that he took for reviews and for himself. Piles of his papers and notes lie on surfaces all around the apartment, some of which were taken from his suitcase that I brought back from Houston. At any time I can peruse our library or his notes and rediscover and recover him.

When I do, I hear him, and he has the last word. Time after time, Christopher has the last word.

June 2012
Washington, D.C.

ABOUT THE AUTHOR

CHRISTOPHER HITCHENS was born April 13, 1949, in England and graduated from Balliol College at Oxford University. The father of three children, he was the author of more than twenty books and pamphlets, including collections of essays, criticism, and reportage. His book *God Is Not Great: How Religon Poisons Everything* was a finalist for the 2007 National Book Award and an international bestseller. His best-selling memoir, *Hitch-22*, was a finalist for the 2010 National Book Critics Circle Award for autobiography. His 2011 bestselling omnibus of selected essays, *Arguably*, was named by the *New York Times* as one of the ten best books of the year. A visiting professor of liberal studies at the New School in New York City, he was also the I. F. Stone professor at the Graduate School of Journalism at the University of California, Berkeley. He was a columnist, literary critic, and contributing editor at *Vanity Fair,* the *Atlantic, Slate,* the *Times Literary Supplement,* the *Nation,* the *New Statesman, World Affairs,* and *Free Inquiry,* among other publications. He died in Houston on December 15, 2011.

MORTALITY

Designed and typeset by Jouve, Brattleboro, Vermont; and Chennai, India

Printed and bound by RR Donnelly, Crawfordsville, Indiana

Composed in Janson MT, a seventeenth-century serif typeface revived in the 1930s by Chauncey H. Griffith; and Requiem Text, a typeface designed by Jonathan Hoefler in 1992 based on inscriptional capitals dating from the 1530s.

ABOUT TWELVE

TWELVE

TWELVE was established in August 2005 with the objective of publishing no more than twelve books each year. We strive to publish the singular book, by authors who have a unique perspective and compelling authority. Works that explain our culture; that illuminate, inspire, provoke, and entertain. We seek to establish communities of conversation surrounding our books. Talented authors deserve attention not only from publishers, but from readers as well. To sell the book is only the beginning of our mission. To build avid audiences of readers who are enriched by these works—that is our ultimate purpose.

For more information about forthcoming TWELVE books, please go to www.twelvebooks.com.